Table of Contents

PREVIEW

Gastrointestinal diseases are among the most common problems in tropical countries and commonly manifest as diarrhea, abdominal pain, abdominal distention, gastrointestinal bleeding, intestinal obstruction, malabsorption, or malnutrition. Infectious diarrheal diseases are an important cause of morbidity and mortality in childhood. This chapter covers acute and chronic diarrheal syndromes, as well as a range of illnesses that affect the mouth, esophagus, stomach, hepatobiliary, and pancreatic systems; small and large bowel; and rectum and anus. Special attention is paid to illnesses more common in the tropics, including duodenal ulcer, gastrointestinal infections, tuberculosis of the abdomen and intestine, malabsorption, tropical enteropathy, tropical sprue, chronic calcific pancreatitis, Helicobacter infection, and intestinal intussusception. Improvement in sanitation and improving socioeconomic conditions have reduced the burden of many infectious diseases, but is associated with an emergence of previously uncommon diseases in the tropics such as inflammatory bowel diseases and celiac disease.

BREAKFAST

1. Veggie Breakfast Sandwich

Prep Time: 15 Minutes

Cook Time: 5 Minutes

Servings: 1

Ingredients

- 1 whole wheat English muffin, sliced in half and toasted (or two fairly small slices of bread, toasted)
- 2 teaspoons mayonnaise
- ½ ripe avocado, mashed
- Salt and freshly ground black pepper
- 1 large egg
- ½ teaspoon water
- 1 teaspoon butter or olive oil
- 2 small slices of cheddar or Monterey Jack cheese (about ½ ounce, any other melty cheese will do)
- 1 slice of ripe red tomato, if tomatoes are in season (optional)

- Thinly sliced red onion

- Several dashes of hot sauce (like Tabasco or Cholula)

- Small handful arugula or sprouts

Instructions

1. To prepare your sandwiches, spread the mayonnaise over the lower half of your toasted muffin. Spread the mashed avocado over the other half, and sprinkle it with a few dashes of salt and pepper.

2. Heat a medium non-stick skillet or well-seasoned cast iron skillet over medium-high heat. In a bowl, scramble the egg with the water and a few dashes of salt and pepper.

3. Once the skillet is hot, add a pat of butter and swirl the pan to coat the bottom. Pour in the scrambled egg and immediately swirl the egg in the bottom of the pan to make an even layer.

4. Immediately place your cheese in the center of the egg mixture as shown. Once the egg is set enough to fold over onto itself with a spatula (this could take 30 seconds to 1 minute), fold one side over the middle, then the opposite side over the middle. Repeat with the other two sides so you have a cute little egg and

cheese envelope. Let it cook for another 15 to 30 seconds, until it's set enough that you can transfer it to a plate.

5. Place the cooked egg on the mayo-covered bun. Top with a slice of tomato, if using. Add with several slices of red onion, a few dashes of hot sauce, and a little handful of arugula. Top it with the remaining bun, avocado side down.

6. To slice it in half, insert a sharp knife into the center of the sandwich, and slice across to one edge. Repeat in the opposite direction. Serve warm! If you're making more sandwiches, reduce the stove temperature from medium-high to medium, as the pan only gets hotter the longer it's on the stove.

Prep Time: 20 Minutes

Cook Time: 15 Minutes

Servings: 12

Ingredients

- 2 cups fresh cranberries
- 2 cups white whole wheat flour or regular whole wheat flour
- 1 teaspoon baking powder
- ½ teaspoon baking soda
- ½ teaspoon fine sea salt
- ⅓ cup melted coconut oil or extra-virgin olive oil
- ¾ cup honey or maple syrup
- 2 eggs, preferably at room temperature
- 1 cup plain Greek yogurt
- 2 teaspoons vanilla extract
- Zest from 1 medium orange (about 1 teaspoon), preferably organic
- 1 tablespoon turbinado sugar (also called raw sugar), for sprinkling on top

Instructions

1. Preheat the oven to 400 degrees Fahrenheit. Grease all 12 cups of your muffin tin or line them with papers, if necessary.

2. In a food processor, process the cranberries for about 5 seconds, until they are broken into little bits (but not puréed—see photos). Set aside.

3. In a large mixing bowl, combine the flour, baking powder, baking soda, and salt. Stir to combine.

4. In a medium mixing bowl, combine the oil and honey and beat together with a whisk. Add the eggs and whisk to combine, then add the yogurt, vanilla and orange zest. Mix well.

5. Pour the wet ingredients into the dry and mix with a big spoon, just until combined (a few lumps are ok). Gently fold the cranberry pieces into the batter.

6. Divide the batter evenly between the 12 muffin cups (they will be quite full). Sprinkle the tops of the muffins with turbinado sugar. Bake the muffins for 15 to 18 minutes, or until the muffins are golden on top and a toothpick inserted into a muffin comes out clean.

7. Place the muffin tin on a cooling rack to cool. You might need to run a butter knife along the outer edge

of the muffins to loosen them from the pan. If you have leftover muffins, store them, covered, at room temperature for 2 days, or in the refrigerator for up to 5 days. Freeze leftover muffins for up to 3 months.

Prep Time: 10 Minutes

Cook Time: 25 Minutes

Servings: 8

Ingredients

- 4 cups old-fashioned rolled oats (use certified gluten-free oats for gluten-free granola)
- 1 ½ cup raw nuts and/or seeds (I used 1 cup pecans and ½ cup pepitas)
- 1 teaspoon fine-grain sea salt (if you're using standard table salt, scale back to ¾ teaspoon)
- ½ teaspoon ground cinnamon
- ½ cup melted coconut oil or olive oil
- ½ cup maple syrup or honey
- 1 teaspoon vanilla extract
- ⅔ cup dried fruit, chopped if large (I used dried cranberries)
- Totally optional additional mix-ins: ½ cup chocolate chips or coconut flakes

Instructions

1. Preheat oven to 350 degrees Fahrenheit and line a large, rimmed baking sheet with parchment paper.
2. In a large mixing bowl, combine the oats, nuts and/or seeds, salt and cinnamon. Stir to blend.
3. Pour in the oil, maple syrup and/or honey and vanilla. Mix well, until every oat and nut is lightly coated. Pour the granola onto your prepared pan and use a large spoon to spread it in an even layer.
4. Bake until lightly golden, about 21 to 24 minutes, stirring halfway (for extra-clumpy granola, press the stirred granola down with your spatula to create a more even layer). The granola will further crisp up as it cools.
5. Let the granola cool completely, undisturbed (at least 45 minutes). Top with the dried fruit (and optional chocolate chips, if using). Break the granola into pieces with your hands if you want to retain big chunks, or stir it around with a spoon if you don't want extra-clumpy granola.
6. Store the granola in an airtight container at room temperature for 1 to 2 weeks, or in a sealed freezer bag in the freezer for up to 3 months. The dried fruit can

freeze solid, so let it warm to room temperature for 5 to 10 minutes before serving.

Prep Time: 20 Minutes

Cook Time: 55 Minutes

Servings: 4

Ingredients

- 2 pounds small-to-medium red or yellow potatoes
- 1 tablespoon plus ¼ teaspoon fine sea salt, divided
- 4 tablespoons olive oil, divided
- ¼ teaspoon garlic powder
- ¼ teaspoon onion powder
- Freshly ground black pepper, to taste
- 2 tablespoons chopped fresh parsley, chives and/or green onion

Instructions

1. To prepare the potatoes, scrub them clean if dirty and rinse under running water. Remove and discard any nubby sprouting areas. Place the potatoes in a large Dutch oven or soup pot.

2. Fill the pot with water until the potatoes are submerged and covered by 1 inch of additional water. Add 1 tablespoon of the salt. Bring the mixture to a boil over medium-high heat and continue cooking until the potatoes are very easily pierced through by a fork (smaller potatoes are done around 20 minutes, and medium around 25 minutes).

3. While the potatoes cook, preheat the oven to 425 degrees Fahrenheit and drizzle 1 tablespoon of the olive oil over a large, rimmed baking sheet. Brush the oil so it's evenly distributed over the sheet.

4. When the potatoes are done, drain them in a large colander and let them cool for about 5 minutes, until they can be handled safely.

5. Evenly distribute the potatoes over the prepared baking sheet, and use a potato masher or a serving fork to gently smash each potato to a height of about ½ inch. (Thinner potatoes are more crispy.)

6. Drizzle the remaining 3 tablespoons of olive oil over the smashed potatoes. Sprinkle the garlic powder, onion powder and remaining ¼ teaspoon salt over the potatoes. Finally, sprinkle them lightly with freshly ground black pepper.

7. Bake until the potatoes are nice and golden on the edges, about 25 to 30 minutes. Sprinkle them with chopped fresh herbs, and serve hot.

Prep Time: 15 Minutes

Cook Time: 15 Minutes

Servings: 4

Ingredients

- 4 small flour or corn tortillas
- 4 large eggs
- 1 tablespoon sour cream (or milk), plus more for serving if desired
- Two dashes of hot sauce, such as Cholula, plus more for serving if desired
- ½ teaspoon fine sea salt, divided
- 1 ½ tablespoons unsalted butter, divided
- 2 cups thinly sliced vegetables (I used a mix of purple cabbage, red bell pepper and carrot)
- ¼ teaspoon chili powder
- ¼ teaspoon ground cumin
- ¼ cup shredded or crumbled cheese, optional (cheddar, Cotijah, feta, goat, even mozzarella)
- ¼ cup thinly sliced green onion

- Suggested garnishes (choose a few): Chopped fresh cilantro, hot sauce or salsa or pico de gallo, strips of avocado or guacamole, diced tomato or sliced cherry tomatoes, sour cream

Instructions

1. Warm the tortillas: You can do this in a large skillet over medium heat in batches, flipping to warm each side. Alternatively, you can warm them directly over a low flame on a gas range. Or, just microwave them in a stack for about 15 to 20 seconds. Stack the warmed tortillas and wrap them with a tea towel to keep warm.
2. Crack the eggs into a bowl and whisk with a fork until the mixture is combined and pure yellow. Add the sour cream or milk, a couple dashes of hot sauce, and ¼ teaspoon of the salt. Whisk to combine, then place the bowl near the stove for later.
3. In a large skillet, melt 1 tablespoon of the butter over medium heat. Add the vegetables, the remaining ¼ teaspoon salt, and the chili powder and cumin. Stir to combine, and cook, stirring occasionally, until the vegetables are tender throughout (about 5 minutes), dialing down the heat to medium-low after a few

minutes have passed. Once cooked, transfer the
vegetables to a bowl and set aside.

4. Return the skillet to the stove over medium-low heat,
    and melt the remaining ½ tablespoon butter. Pour in
    the egg mixture. Use a spatula to gently stir and push
    the eggs around the skillet until the eggs are clumpy
    but still slightly wet, about 3 to 5 minutes.

5. Remove the skillet from the heat. Add the cheese (if
    using) and green onion, and gently stir to combine.

6. Assemble your tacos by spooning scrambled eggs
    down the length of a tortilla, topping with some
    cooked veggies, and your garnishes of choice. Enjoy
    warm. Leftover tacos will keep fairly well in the
    refrigerator for up to 4 days; gently reheat before
    serving.

Prep Time: 30 Minutes

Cook Time: 15 Minutes

Servings: 8

Ingredients

- 8 corn tortillas (make sure they're 100% corn or they won't get crispy)
- 1 tablespoon extra-virgin olive oil
- 2 cups refried beans, warmed
- ½ cup grated sharp cheddar cheese
- 8 eggs, fried or scrambled (your preference)
- 2 cups pico de gallo
- Optional garnishes, for serving: your favorite hot sauce or salsa, avocado, and/or crumbled Cotijah or feta cheese

Instructions

1. To prepare the crispy tortillas: Preheat the oven to 400 degrees Fahrenheit with two racks placed near the middle of the oven. Line two large rimmed baking

sheets with parchment paper for easy cleanup, if you'd like.

2. On the baking sheets, brush both sides of each tortilla lightly with oil. Arrange 4 tortillas in a single layer across each pan. Bake for 10 to 12 minutes, turning halfway, until each tortilla is golden and lightly crisp. Set aside.

3. Meanwhile, prepare the remaining components (refried beans, pico de gallo, and eggs, cooked to your liking).

4. To assemble, spread warm refried beans over each tostada. Top with a sprinkle of cheese, cooked egg(s) and use a slotted spoon or serving fork to top the eggs with pico de gallo. Top with any optional garnishes you'd like, and serve promptly.

5. Tostadas are best enjoyed fresh, since the tortillas will lose their crispness with time. However, the leftovers are still good to me! They'll keep for about 3 days in the refrigerator. If you have leftover refried beans and/or pico de gallo, they both make a great dip for tortilla chips or filling for quesadillas or burritos.

Prep Time: 15 Minutes

Cook Time: 15 Minutes

Servings: 4

Ingredients

- 8 large eggs
- ⅓ cup whole milk or milk of choice
- Pinch of fine sea salt
- Freshly ground black pepper
- 1 tablespoon unsalted butter
- 3 cups baby spinach, roughly chopped
- 4 ounces goat cheese, crumbled (about 1 cup)
- ½ cup chopped green onion, mostly green parts
- ⅓ cup oil-packed sun-dried tomatoes, rinsed and roughly chopped
- Optional, for serving: flaky sea salt for sprinkling on top, toasted whole-grain bread

Instructions

1. Crack the eggs into a large bowl. Add the milk, salt and about 10 twists of black pepper. Whisk until the mixture is thoroughly combined and pure yellow. Be sure to have your remaining ingredients prepped and ready, because this recipe comes together quickly once you start cooking.

2. Warm a medium skillet over medium heat. Add the butter and let it melt.

3. Add the spinach and cook, stirring with a silicone or rubber spatula, until the spinach is wilted and bright green, about 1 to 2 minutes.

4. Pour the eggs into the skillet and reduce the heat to medium-low. Use your spatula to gently stir and push the eggs around the skillet until the eggs are clumpy but still slightly wet, about 3 to 5 minutes.

5. Remove the skillet from the heat. Add the goat cheese, green onion and sun-dried tomatoes, and gently stir to combine. Divide the mixture into bowls. Sprinkle lightly with optional flaky sea salt, and serve with toast if you'd like. Serve promptly.

Prep Time: 25 Minutes

Cook Time: 30 Minutes

Servings: 6

Ingredients

- Six 8" whole grain tortillas
- 1 full batch homemade hash browns
- 6 large eggs
- 1 cup cooked pinto beans or black beans (I used canned beans, rinsed and drained)
- ¼ teaspoon salt
- Several dashes of hot sauce, such as Cholula
- 1 tablespoon unsalted butter
- ⅔ cup (packed) shredded sharp cheddar cheese
- ½ cup chopped cilantro, divided
- ½ cup chopped green onion (mostly green parts), divided
- 6 tablespoons of your favorite salsa, plus extra for serving
- 1 large avocado, diced (optional, if you're serving the burritos right away)

Instructions

1. To prepare the eggs: Crack the eggs into a medium bowl and whisk them with a fork until the mixture is pale yellow. Stir in the beans and season with the salt and hot sauce.

2. To cook the eggs: Melt the butter in a medium-sized skillet (either well-seasoned cast iron or nonstick) over medium heat. Pour in the egg mixture and cook, stirring often, until the eggs are just set, about 2 to 4 minutes. Stir in the cheese and transfer the mixture to a bowl. Then stir in the cilantro and green onion (if you're serving the burritos right away, reserve a small amount of each for garnish).

3. To make sure the tortillas are nice and pliable, quickly run each tortilla under running water (trust me). Warm the tortillas briefly in the microwave (about 10 to 20 seconds) or in a skillet.

4. Working with one tortilla at a time, spread about ⅓ cup hash browns on a tortilla about one-third from the edge. Drizzle 1 tablespoon salsa on top of the hash browns. Top with about cup scrambled eggs. (You can eyeball the amounts of hash browns and scrambled eggs; just try to divide them evenly between the tortillas.)

5. Roll up the burrito by first folding the tortilla over from the bottom to partially cover the contents, then fold in the two sides. Finish rolling and put the burrito seam side down on a plate. Repeat with the remaining burritos.

6. If you're serving the burritos right away: You can halve the burritos like I did, or serve them whole. Warm some extra salsa in the microwave or on the stove, then pour it over the burritos. Top with diced avocado (if using) and the reserved cilantro and green onion. Serve immediately, with a knife and a fork.

7. If you're freezing the burritos for later: Let the burritos cool to room temperature, then wrap each burrito in plastic wrap. Transfer the wrapped burritos to a freezer-safe bag and squeeze out the air before sealing. Store the burritos in the freezer. For best flavor, consume your burritos within 3 to 6 months.

8. To defrost frozen burritos, unwrap the plastic wrap and then wrap the burrito in a damp paper towel. Microwave about 2 to 3 minutes, until warmed throughout. I like to serve mine with some extra salsa.

Prep Time: 15 Minutes

Cook Time: 15 Minutes

Servings: 4

Ingredients

- 1 pound Russet potatoes (2 small-to-medium), peeled if desired
- ½ teaspoon salt
- ¼ teaspoon garlic powder
- ¼ teaspoon onion powder
- ¼ cup extra-virgin olive oil

Instructions

1. Scrub the potatoes clean and grate them on a large-holed cheese grater (I left the skin on, but you can peel it first if you'd like). In a fine-mesh sieve, rinse the grated potato well until the water runs clear.
2. Drain the potatoes, and then place them potato on a clean tea towel or several paper towels. Twist the

towel to remove as much moisture from the potatoes as possible (you might need to do this in two batches).

3. Transfer the grated potato to a bowl and toss it with the salt, garlic powder and onion powder.

4. In a large skillet (preferably cast iron, but non-stick works, too), warm the olive oil over medium heat until shimmering and a piece of grated potato sizzles on contact. Spread the potatoes over the skillet in an even layer and press them down with a spatula. Let them cook, undisturbed, for 2 minutes.

5. Stir again, press them down again, and cook for another 2 minutes. Repeat in 2-minute intervals, flipping in sections once they're crispy enough to do so, until the potatoes are golden brown and crispy, about 4 to 8 more minutes. Meanwhile, line a plate with a couple of layers of paper towels to absorb excess oil, and set it near the stove.

6. Transfer the hash browns to the lined plate and let them drain for a minute. (If you're making multiply batches of hash browns, repeat these steps as necessary—keep in mind that your skillet will be really hot so your next batch may cook faster.)

7. Season to taste with additional salt, if necessary, and serve hot.

Prep Time: 10 Minutes

Cook Time: 20 Minutes

Servings: 8

Ingredients

- 2 teaspoons orange zest (from about 1 ½ oranges, preferably organic)
- 2 tablespoons sugar
- 4 cups old-fashioned rolled oats
- 1 ½ cup raw almonds
- 1 teaspoon fine sea salt (if you're using standard table salt, scale back to ¾ teaspoon)
- 1 teaspoon ground cinnamon
- ½ cup extra-virgin olive oil or melted coconut oil
- ½ cup honey or maple syrup
- 1 tablespoon vanilla extract
- ¾ cup raisins, preferably golden

Instructions

1. Preheat the oven to 350 degrees Fahrenheit and line a large, rimmed baking sheet with parchment paper.

2. In a small bowl, combine the orange zest and sugar. Use your fingers to rub the zest into the sugar until it's bright orange and very fragrant. This step will ensure that your granola is infused with orange flavor.

3. In a large mixing bowl, combine the oats, almonds, salt, cinnamon and orange sugar. Stir to combine. Pour in the olive oil, honey and vanilla, and mix well.

4. Pour the granola onto your prepared baking sheet. Spread the granola into an even layer. Bake for 19 to 23 minutes, stirring halfway, until the granola is turning lightly golden in color. The granola will crisp up as it cools.

5. Let the granola cool before stirring in the raisins and breaking up the granola into chunks as necessary. Store the granola in an airtight container at room temperature for 1 to 2 weeks, or keep it in the freezer for longer shelf life.

11. Tangy Lentil Salad with Dill & Pepperoncini

Prep Time: 25 Minutes

Cook Time: 20 Minutes

Servings: 4-6

Ingredients

Salad:

- 1 ½ cups black beluga lentils
- 1 bay leaf
- ½ teaspoon fine sea salt
- 2 cups grated carrots (about ¾ pound or 5 to 6 medium carrots, peeled and grated on the large holes of a box grater or in a food processor fitted with a grating attachment)
- ¾ cup fresh flat-leaf parsley
- ¼ cup (⅓ ounce) fresh dill leaves, tough stems removed, torn into small pieces
- ½ cup chopped celery (about 2 ribs)
- ½ cup thinly sliced green onion
- ½ cup chopped pickled pepperoncini pepper

- Optional cheese: ½ cup tiny cubes of havarti, havarti dill, mild cheddar, or crumbled feta

Tahini-dill dressing:

- ⅓ cup extra-virgin olive oil
- ¼ cup lemon juice
- ¼ cup (⅓ ounce) fresh dill leaves, tough stems removed
- 2 tablespoons tahini
- 1 clove garlic, roughly chopped
- ½ teaspoon fine sea salt, to taste
- ½ teaspoon red pepper flakes (scale back or omit if sensitive to spice), to taste
- Freshly ground black pepper, to taste

Instructions

1. To cook the lentils: Fill a medium-to-large saucepan with water, leaving several inches of room at the top. Bring it to a boil over high heat.
2. Meanwhile, sort through your lentils for debris, then rinse your lentils in a fine-mesh sieve under running water until the water runs clear. Set aside.

3. Once the water is boiling, add the rinsed lentils. Add the bay leaf and salt. Set the timer for 16 minutes. Reduce the heat as necessary to prevent overflow and to maintain a lively simmer.

4. Meanwhile, make the dressing in a food processor: Combine the olive oil, lemon juice, dill, tahini, garlic, salt, red pepper flakes and several twists of black pepper. Blend until smooth, pausing to scrape down the sides and the bottom of the bowl as necessary. Set aside.

5. Once your timer has gone off, use a fork to scoop out a few lentils and test for doneness (careful, they're hot). Your lentils are done when they are pleasantly tender throughout (not mushy or falling apart) and taste nicely earthy (undercooked lentils tend to taste somewhat metallic). If your lentils aren't fully cooked yet, retest every 1 to 2 minutes until they are. Once cooked, strain off all the excess water.

6. Pour the lentils into a medium serving bowl, and discard the bay leaf. Pour in all of the dressing, and stir to combine. Add the grated carrots, parsley, the remaining dill, celery, green onion, and pepperoncini peppers. Wait to add the optional cheese until the

lentils are just warm (not hot enough to melt the cheese).

7. Stir to combine. Season to taste with additional salt (for overall flavor), red pepper flakes (for heat) and/or black pepper. If the salad isn't tangy enough for your liking, you could add a tablespoon more lemon juice or chopped pepperoncinis.

8. This salad is ready to serve, though it tastes even better after a 20-minute rest. It keeps well in the refrigerator, covered, for about 4 days.

Prep Time: 25 Minutes

Cook Time: 15 Minutes

Servings: 6

Ingredients

- 8 ounces soba noodles or spaghetti noodles of choice
- ¼ cup raw sesame seeds
- ⅓ cup reduced sodium tamari (or soy sauce, just be sure it's reduced sodium or it will taste too salty)
- ¼ cup toasted sesame oil
- 2 tablespoons lime juice (about 1 medium lime)
- 1 teaspoon grated fresh ginger
- 2 cloves garlic, pressed or minced
- ½ teaspoon red pepper flakes, to taste (scale back or omit if sensitive to spice)
- 2 ½ cups thinly sliced red cabbage (about 10 ounces or ¼th medium cabbage)
- 3 whole carrots, peeled and then sliced into ribbons with vegetable peeler (about 1 ½ cups)
- 1 red bell pepper, sliced into very thin strips
- 1 bunch green onions, chopped

- ½ cup chopped cilantro
- Optional: 2 cups shelled edamame, steamed

Instructions

1. Cook the soba noodles according to the package directions. Once they're done cooking, drain them in a colander and rinse them well under cool water. Transfer the drained noodles to a large serving bowl and set aside.

2. Meanwhile, toast the sesame seeds in a small skillet over medium heat, stirring often (keep an eye on them, as they can burn quickly). Once they're fragrant and turning golden, transfer them to a small bowl so they don't burn. Set aside.

3. In another bowl, combine the tamari, sesame oil, lime juice, ginger, garlic and red pepper flakes. Whisk until blended. Set aside.

4. To assemble, add the cabbage, carrots, bell pepper, green onions, cilantro and optional edamame to your bowl with the noodles. Drizzle in the dressing. Add all of the sesame seeds, and use tongs to toss until the mixture is fully combined. Serve immediately, or refrigerate for later. This salad is best consumed

within a couple of days, but it will keep for up to 5 days.

Prep Time: 15 Minutes

Cook Time: 30 Minutes

Servings: 4

Ingredients

Roasted cauliflower:

- 1 large head cauliflower (about 2 pounds), cut into bite-sized florets
- 2 tablespoons extra-virgin olive oil
- ¼ teaspoon red pepper flakes (scale back or omit if sensitive to spice)
- ¼ teaspoon fine sea salt
- Garlicky faro:
- 1 cup uncooked farro, rinsed
- 2 teaspoons extra-virgin olive oil
- 2 cloves garlic, pressed or minced
- ¼ teaspoon fine sea salt

Everything else:

- ⅓ cup pitted Kalamata olives, rinsed, half sliced into small rounds and the rest halved lengthwise

- ¼ cup oil-packed sun-dried tomatoes, rinsed and roughly chopped
- ½ cup crumbled feta (about 2 ounces)
- 1 tablespoon lemon juice (about ½ lemon), plus more for serving
- Freshly ground black pepper, to taste
- 1 avocado, sliced into thin strips
- 4+ handfuls leafy greens (spring greens, spinach, arugula or baby kale are all good choices)

Instructions

1. To roast the cauliflower: Preheat the oven to 425 degrees Fahrenheit. Toss the cauliflower florets with the olive oil, red pepper flakes and salt, and arrange it in an even layer across the pan. Roast for 25 to 35 minutes, tossing halfway, until the cauliflower is tender and deeply golden on the edges.

2. To cook the farro: In a medium saucepan, combine the rinsed farro with at least three cups water (enough water to cover the farro by a couple of inches). Bring the water to a boil, then reduce the heat to a gentle simmer, and cook until the farro is tender to the bite but still pleasantly chewy. (Pearled farro will take

around 15 minutes; unprocessed farro will take 25 to 40 minutes.) Drain off the excess water and mix in the olive oil, garlic and salt. Set aside.

3. In a large serving bowl, toss together the roasted cauliflower, cooked farro, olives, sun-dried tomatoes, feta and lemon juice. Taste and season with additional salt and pepper if necessary.

4. Divide the avocado and greens between four dinner plates. Top with a generous amount of the cauliflower and farro salad. Finish the plates with an extra squeeze of lemon juice or drizzle of olive oil, if desired. Serve promptly.

Prep Time: 30 Minutes

Cook Time: 45 Minutes

Servings: 4

Ingredients

Crispy baked tofu and rice:

- 1 block (12 to 15 ounces) organic extra-firm tofu
- 1 tablespoon extra-virgin olive oil
- 1 tablespoon reduced-sodium tamari or soy sauce
- 1 tablespoon cornstarch or arrowroot starch
- 1 ¼ cups brown basmati rice or long-grain brown rice, rinsed

Peanut sauce:

- ⅓ cup creamy peanut butter
- 3 tablespoons lime juice (about 1 lime)
- 2 tablespoons reduced-sodium tamari or soy sauce
- 1 tablespoon honey or maple syrup, to taste
- 2 teaspoons toasted sesame oil
- 2 garlic cloves, pressed or minced

- ¼ teaspoon red pepper flakes (omit or reduce if sensitive to spice)
- Mango salsa and cabbage:
- 2 large ripe mangos, diced
- 1 medium red bell pepper, chopped
- ½ cup (about 4) thinly sliced green onions
- ¼ cup chopped fresh cilantro
- 1 medium jalapeño, seeds and ribs removed, minced
- 2 tablespoons lime juice
- ¼ teaspoon fine sea salt
- 2 cups shredded purple or green cabbage
- Handful of chopped roasted peanuts, for garnish

Instructions

1. Preheat the oven to 400 degrees Fahrenheit and line a large, rimmed baking sheet with parchment paper to prevent the tofu from sticking.
2. To prepare the tofu: Drain the tofu and use your palms to gently squeeze out some of the water. Slice the tofu into thirds lengthwise so you have 3 even slabs. Stack the slabs on top of each other and slice through them lengthwise to make 3 even columns, then slice across to make 5 even rows.

3. Line a cutting board with a lint-free tea towel or paper
    towels, then arrange the tofu in an even layer on the
    towel(s). Fold the towel(s) over the cubed tofu, then
    place something heavy on top (like another cutting
    board, topped with a cast iron pan or large cans of
    tomatoes) to help the tofu drain. Let the tofu rest for
    at least 10 minutes (preferably more like 30 minutes,
    if you have the time).

4. Meanwhile, bring a large pot of water to boil. Add the
    rice and boil, uncovered, for 30 minutes. Drain off the
    remaining cooking water and return the rice to the
    pot. Cover the pot and let the rice rest, off the heat, for
    10 minutes. Fluff with a fork and set aside.

5. Transfer the pressed tofu to the lined baking sheet
    and drizzle with the olive oil and tamari. Toss to
    combine. Sprinkle the starch over the tofu, and toss
    the tofu until the starch is evenly coated, so there are
    no powdery spots remaining.

6. Arrange the tofu in an even layer. Bake for 25 to 30
    minutes, tossing the tofu halfway, until the tofu is
    deeply golden on the edges. Set aside.

7. Meanwhile, prepare the peanut sauce by whisking all
    the ingredients together in a bowl. Taste, and if it's too

bold, add another teaspoon of honey to tame it. Set aside.

8. Then, in a medium mixing bowl, combine the diced mango, bell pepper, green onion, cilantro, jalapeño, lime juice and salt. Stir to combine, and set aside.

9. To assemble your bowls, start with a big scoop of cooked rice. Top with a handful (½ cup) shredded cabbage, then a big scoop of mango salsa, a handful of baked tofu, a hefty drizzle of peanut sauce, and a little sprinkle of chopped peanuts. Leftover bowls will keep well in the refrigerator, covered, for about 4 days.

Prep Time: 15 Minutes

Cook Time: 45 Minutes

Servings: 4

Ingredients

Salad:

- 1 cup wild rice, rinsed
- ½ cup sliced almonds
- 1 teaspoon olive oil
- 5 ounces arugula (about 5 packed cups)
- ½ cup coarsely chopped fresh basil (from one ⅔ ounce container)
- ½ cup dried tart cherries or cranberries, chopped
- ½ cup crumbled feta or goat cheese (about 2 ounces)

Lemon dressing:

- ¼ cup olive oil
- 2 tablespoons lemon juice (from 1 medium lemon), to taste
- 2 teaspoons Dijon mustard
- 1 teaspoon honey or maple syrup

- 1 medium clove garlic, pressed or minced

- ¼ teaspoon fine sea salt, to taste

- Freshly ground black pepper, to taste

Instructions

1. To cook the wild rice, bring a large pot of water to boil. Add the rinsed rice and continue boiling, reducing heat as necessary to prevent overflow, for 40 minutes to 55 minutes, until the rice is pleasantly tender but still offers a light resistance to the bite. Remove from heat, drain the rice and return the rice to pot. Cover and let the rice rest for 10 minutes, then remove the lid and let the rice cool.

2. To toast the almonds, warm one teaspoon olive oil in a small skillet over medium-low heat. Add the almonds and a pinch of salt and cook until they're turning lightly golden and fragrant, about 4 to 5 minutes, stirring frequently. Set aside to cool.

3. In a small bowl, whisk together the dressing ingredients until blended.

4. To assemble the salad, transfer the cooled rice to a large bowl. Add the arugula, chopped basil, almonds, sour cherries and feta. Pour in the dressing, toss well,

and season to taste with additional salt (I usually add another pinch or two) and pepper. If the salad needs more fresh, bright flavor, add up to 1 tablespoon more lemon juice.

5. Set the salad aside for 10 minutes before serving, to give the rice time to soak up some of the dressing. This salad keeps well in the refrigerator, covered, for two to three days. You might need to wake up leftovers with an extra drizzle of olive oil and squeeze of lemon (the rice absorbs the dressing over time).

Prep Time: 20 Minutes

Cook Time: 25 Minutes

Servings: 4

Ingredients

Carrot salad:

- 1 pound carrots, peeled
- 2 tablespoons finely snipped chives or chopped green onion
- 2 tablespoons finely chopped fresh parsley
- Optional: 1 can (15 ounces) chickpeas, rinsed and drained, or 1 ½ cups cooked chickpeas

Dressing:

- 2 tablespoons extra-virgin olive oil
- 2 tablespoons lemon juice
- 2 teaspoons honey
- 1 teaspoon Dijon mustard
- ½ teaspoon ground cumin
- ¼ teaspoon fine sea salt

Instructions

1. To prepare the carrots: You can grate them on the large holes of a box grater, or use short strokes with a julienne peeler, or process them in a food processor fitted with a grating attachment. You'll end up with about 3 cups grated carrots.
2. Place the carrots in a medium serving bowl. Add the chives, parsley and optional chickpeas to the bowl.
3. To make the dressing, whisk all of the ingredients together in a small bowl until completely blended.
4. Pour the dressing over the carrot mixture and stir until the mixture is evenly coated in dressing. For best flavor, allow the salad to marinate for 20 minutes before serving. Toss again before serving. This salad keeps well in the refrigerator, covered, for about 4 days.

Prep Time: 20 Minutes

Cook Time: 25 Minutes

Servings: 4

Ingredients

Salad:

- 1 cup uncooked farro, rinsed
- ¼ teaspoon fine sea salt
- 1 big bunch curly green kale, ribs removed and chopped into small, bite-sized pieces
- ½ cup raw sliced almonds
- ⅓ cup roughly chopped dried cherries or cranberries
- 4 ounces goat cheese, crumbled

Vinaigrette:

- ⅓ cup extra-virgin olive oil
- 1 tablespoon + 1 teaspoon sherry vinegar or red wine vinegar
- 1 tablespoon Dijon mustard
- 2 cloves garlic, pressed or minced
- ¼ teaspoon fine sea salt

Instructions

1. To cook the farro, in a medium saucepan, combine the rinsed farro with at least three cups water (enough water to cover the farro by a couple of inches). Add the salt, bring the water to a boil, then reduce the heat to maintain a gentle simmer. Cook until the farro is tender to the bite but still pleasantly chewy. (Pearled farro will take around 15 minutes; unprocessed farro will take 25 to 40 minutes.) Drain off the excess water and set aside.

2. Meanwhile, place the chopped kale in a large serving bowl. Sprinkle it with a few dashes of salt and massage it with your hands by scrunching up large handfuls at a time until it's darker and more fragrant (this makes the kale taste less bitter and makes it easier to eat). Set aside.

3. To toast the almonds, pour them into a small skillet. Cook over medium heat, stirring frequently (careful, they can burn), until the almonds are fragrant and starting to turn golden on the edges, about 4 to 5 minutes. Pour the almonds into the bowl of massaged kale.

4. To prepare the vinaigrette, simply whisk the ingredients together in a liquid measuring cup or small bowl. Set aside.

5. Once the farro has been cooked and drained, stir in the chopped dried cherries (so they have a chance to plump up a bit) and vinaigrette (the heat will temper the garlic a bit).

6. Once the farro has cooled down to room temperature or close to it, stir it into the kale mixture. Gently crumble most of the goat cheese into the salad and lightly stir. Taste, and if the salad doesn't taste amazing yet, stir in more vinegar by the teaspoon until it does.

7. Crumble the remaining goat cheese on top of the salad. Serve promptly, or refrigerate for later. This salad keeps well for four to five days in the refrigerator, covered.

Prep Time: 20 Minutes

Cook Time: 1hrs 25 Minutes

Servings: 6-8

Ingredients

Lentils:

- 1 tablespoon olive oil
- 1 red onion, chopped
- ¼ teaspoon salt
- 2 cloves garlic, pressed or minced
- 1 ¼ cups regular brown lentils, picked over for debris and rinsed
- 3 cups water
- Pasta and everything else
- 12 ounces whole grain ziti, rigatoni or penne pasta
- 8 ounces (2 packed cups) grated part-skim mozzarella cheese, divided
- Salt, to taste
- Freshly ground black pepper, to taste
- Pinch of red pepper flakes (omit if sensitive to spice)

- 23.5 ounces Newman's Own Organics Marinara (plus 1 cup extra sauce, if you like extra-saucy ziti like me), divided

- 1 cup cottage cheese or ricotta cheese

- Handful of torn fresh basil leaves, for garnishing

Instructions

1. To cook the lentils: In a large saucepan over medium heat, warm the olive oil until shimmering. Add the onion and salt. Cook, stirring occasionally, until the onion is turning translucent, about 4 to 5 minutes. Add the garlic and cook until fragrant, about 30 seconds. Add the lentils and water, and stir to combine.

2. Raise the heat to high and bring the mixture to a simmer, then reduce heat to medium-low and gently simmer until the lentils are tender and cooked through, about 30 to 40 minutes. Drain the mixture well in a fine-mesh sieve and return the lentils to their pot. Set aside.

3. Meanwhile, preheat the oven to 350 degrees Fahrenheit and bring a large pot of salted water to boil. Cook the pasta just until al dente, according to

package directions. Drain and return the pasta to the pot.

4. Add the lentils to the pasta. Add ½ cup of the cheese, reserving the rest for later. Season to taste with salt (I usually add ¼ to ½ teaspoon), freshly ground black pepper and red pepper flakes (if using).

5. Pour 1 cup of the marinara sauce into a 13×9-inch baking dish. Spread the sauce around with a spatula so the base of the baker is evenly coated. Pour the lentil and pasta mixture into the baker and spread it so it's evenly distributed. Using a spoon, dollop cottage cheese in big spoonfuls over the pasta, then just lightly swirl the mixture a bit so the cottage cheese is still concentrated in those areas.

6. Drizzle the rest of the sauce evenly over the dish (adding extra sauce if you'd like) and gently spread it over the pasta. Sprinkle the remaining mozzarella evenly over the dish. Cover the baker tightly with aluminum foil—don't let it touch the cheese—or stick a few wooden toothpicks down the center and place a generously sized piece of parchment paper, folded in the middle to make a "tent" over the baker.

7. Bake for 30 minutes, then remove the covering, increase the heat to 450, and continue baking until

the cheese on top is golden and spotty, 3 to 9 more minutes. Remove the baker from the oven and let it cool for 10 minutes before serving (trust me). Sprinkle freshly torn basil on top, slice and serve.

Prep Time: 15 Minutes

Cook Time: 60 Minutes

Servings: 6

Ingredients

- 3 tablespoons extra-virgin olive oil, divided
- 1 medium yellow onion, chopped fine
- 1 ½ teaspoons fine sea salt, divided
- 6 garlic cloves, pressed or minced
- 2 teaspoons smoked paprika
- 1 can (15 ounces) diced tomatoes (preferably the fire-roasted variety), drained
- 2 cups short-grain brown rice
- 1 can (15 ounces) chickpeas, rinsed and drained, or 1 ½ cups cooked chickpeas
- 3 cups vegetable broth
- ⅓ cup dry white wine or vegetable broth
- ½ teaspoon saffron threads, crumbled (optional)
- 1 can (14 ounces) quartered artichokes or 1 jar (12 ounces) marinated artichoke, drained

- 2 red bell peppers, stemmed, seeded and sliced into long, ½"-wide strips
- ½ cup Kalamata olives, pitted and halved
- Freshly ground black pepper
- ¼ cup chopped fresh parsley, plus about 1 tablespoon more for garnish
- 2 tablespoons lemon juice, plus additional lemon wedges for garnish
- ½ cup frozen peas

Instructions

1. Arrange your oven racks in the upper and lower thirds of the oven, making sure that you have ample space between the two racks for your Dutch oven. You're going to need a large Dutch oven (preferably 6 quarts/11-to-12" in diameter or bigger, although I got by with my 5.5-quart Le Creuset) or a large skillet with a snug-fitting lid (both must be oven-safe!).

2. Preheat the oven to 350 degrees Fahrenheit. Heat 2 tablespoons of the oil in your Dutch oven or skillet over medium heat until shimmering. Add the onion and a pinch of salt. Cook until the onions are tender and translucent, about 5 minutes.

3. Stir in the garlic and paprika and cook until fragrant, about 30 seconds. Stir in the tomatoes and cook until the mixture begins to darken and thicken slightly, about 2 minutes Stir in the rice and cook until the grains are well coated with tomato mixture, about 1 minute. Stir in the chickpeas, broth, wine, saffron (if using) and 1 teaspoon salt.

4. Increase the heat to medium-high and bring the mixture to a boil, stirring occasionally. Cover the pot and transfer it to the lower rack in the oven. Bake, undisturbed, until the liquid is absorbed and the rice is tender, 50 to 55 minutes.

5. Meanwhile, line a large, rimmed baking sheet with parchment paper for easy cleanup. On the baking sheet, combine the artichoke, peppers, chopped olives, 1 tablespoon of the olive oil, ½ teaspoon of the salt, and about 10 twists of freshly ground black pepper. Toss to combine, then spread the contents evenly across the pan.

6. Roast the vegetables on the upper rack until the artichokes and peppers are tender and browned around the edges, about 40 to 45 minutes. Remove from the oven and let the vegetables cool for a few minutes. Add ¼ cup parsley to the pan and the lemon

juice, and toss to combine. Season with salt and pepper, to taste. Set aside.

7. For optional socarrat (crispy bottom—beware that you might have to scrub burnt bits from your pot later if you do this): Uncover the pot of baked rice, transfer it to the stovetop and cook over medium-high heat for about 5 minutes, rotating the pot as needed, until the bottom layer of rice is well browned and crisp.

8. Socarrat or not, sprinkle the peas and roasted vegetables over the baked rice, cover, and let the paella sit for 5 minutes. Garnish with a sprinkle of chopped parsley (about 1 tablespoon) and serve in individual bowls, with lemon wedges on the side.

20. Orange Orzo Salad with Almonds, Feta and Olives

Prep Time: 15 Minutes

Cook Time: 10 Minutes

Servings: 6

Ingredients

- 8 ounces whole wheat orzo pasta (I used DeLallo brand)
- ½ cup raw almonds
- 1 cup chopped flat-leaf parsley
- ½ cup pitted Kalamata olives, halved
- ½ cup chopped green onion
- ½ cup raisins, preferably golden
- ½ cup crumbled feta cheese (optional)
- 1 teaspoon orange zest
- ¼ cup fresh-squeezed orange juice (from 1 to 2 oranges, preferably organic)
- ¼ cup extra-virgin olive oil
- 2 tablespoons white wine vinegar
- 1 medium clove garlic, pressed or minced
- ¼ teaspoon salt
- Freshly ground black pepper, to taste

Instructions

1. Bring a large pot of salted water to boil. Add the orzo and cook until al dente, according to package directions. Before draining, reserve roughly ½ cup pasta cooking water. Drain, and immediately rinse the orzo under cold running water until the orzo is no longer warm. Drain well.

2. Toast the almonds in a medium skillet over medium heat, stirring frequently, until fragrant and turning golden on the edges, about 5 minutes. Transfer the almonds to a cutting board and chop them.

3. In a large serving bowl, combine the cooked orzo, chopped almonds, parsley, olives, green onion, raisins, and feta (if using).

4. In a liquid measuring cup or small bowl, combine the orange zest, orange juice, olive oil, vinegar, garlic and salt. Add ¼ cup of the reserved pasta cooking water, and whisk until blended.

5. Pour the dressing over the salad and toss to combine. It might seem like too much dressing at first, but don't worry. Season with pepper, to taste.

6. Let the orzo salad rest for at least 10 minutes (or up to several hours in the refrigerator) so it has time to soak up the dressing. Season to taste with additional salt, if

necessary, and serve. Leftovers will keep well in the refrigerator for up to four days.

21. Caprese Pasta Salad

Prep Time: 15 Minutes

Cook Time: 10 Minutes

Servings: 4

Ingredients

- 6 ounces (2 cups) whole grain fusilli or rotini pasta
- ⅓ cup extra-virgin olive oil
- 2 pints cherry or grape tomatoes
- ½ teaspoon fine sea salt
- 8 ounces mozzarella "pearls", or one mozzarella ball, torn into bite-sized pieces
- Several sprigs of fresh basil (enough for 2+ tablespoons chopped)
- 2 to 3 teaspoons white balsamic vinegar or regular balsamic vinegar, to taste

Instructions

1. Bring a large pot of salted water to boil and cook the
    pasta until al dente, according to package
    instructions. Drain the pasta and set it aside.

2. While the pasta is cooking, combine the olive oil,
    tomatoes and salt in a large, non-reactive skillet or
    Dutch oven over medium heat. Cover the skillet (use a
    baking sheet if you don't have a better lid). Cook,
    stirring occasionally, until most of the tomatoes have
    started to burst out of their skins and the olive oil has
    a light red hue (about 6 to 12 minutes).

3. Remove the skillet from the heat and stir in the
    cooked pasta. Let the mixture cool for a few minutes
    while you chop the basil. We don't want the cheese to
    melt on contact, so wait to proceed to the next step
    until your pasta is lightly warm (not hot).

4. Stir the mozzarella balls and basil into the pasta. Add
    the vinegar, then taste and add additional vinegar
    and/or salt, if it doesn't quite taste spectacular yet.
    For best flavor, let the mixture rest for about 20
    minutes, so the pasta can absorb some of the sauce.
    Or, refrigerate it for future use.

5. This salad will keep well in the refrigerator for up to 4
    days. Leftovers are great chilled or at room

temperature. You can also reheat the pasta if you don't mind the mozzarella melting (yum).

Prep Time: 10 Minutes

Cook Time: 50 Minutes

Servings: 4

Ingredients

Roasted spaghetti squash:

- 2 medium spaghetti squash (about 2 pounds each), halved and seeds removed
- 2 tablespoons olive oil
- Salt and freshly ground black pepper
- Cabbage and black bean slaw
- 2 cups purple cabbage, thinly sliced and roughly chopped into 2-inch long pieces
- 1 can (15 ounces) black beans, rinsed and drained
- 1 red bell pepper, chopped
- ⅓ cup chopped green onions, both green and white parts
- ⅓ cup chopped fresh cilantro
- 2 to 3 tablespoons fresh lime juice, to taste
- 1 teaspoon olive oil

- ¼ teaspoon salt

- Avocado salsa verde

- ¾ cup mild salsa verde, either homemade or store-bought

- 1 ripe avocado, diced

- ⅓ cup fresh cilantro (a few stems are ok)

- 1 tablespoon fresh lime juice

- 1 medium garlic clove, roughly chopped

- Optional garnishes: chopped fresh cilantro, crumbled feta and/or seasoned toasted pepitas (not shown)

Instructions

1. To roast the spaghetti squash: Preheat the oven to 400 degrees Fahrenheit and line a large baking sheet with parchment paper for easy clean-up. On the baking sheet, drizzle the halved spaghetti squash with olive oil. Rub the olive oil all over each of the halves, adding more if necessary.

2. Sprinkle the insides of the squash with freshly ground black pepper and salt. Turn them over so the insides are facing down. Roast for 40 to 60 minutes, until the flesh is easily pierced through with a fork.

3. Meanwhile, to assemble the slaw: In a medium mixing bowl, combine the cabbage, black beans, bell pepper, green onion, cilantro, lime juice, olive oil and salt. Toss to combine and set aside to marinate.

4. To make the salsa verde: In the bowl of a blender or food processor, combine the avocado, salsa verde, cilantro, lime juice and garlic. Blend until smooth, pausing to scrape down the sides as necessary.

5. To assemble, first use a fork to separate and fluff up the flesh of the spaghetti squash. Then divide the slaw into each of the spaghetti squash "bowls," and add a big dollop of avocado salsa verde. Finish the bowls with another sprinkle of pepper, cilantro and optional crumbled feta or pepitas.

Prep Time: 20 Minutes

Cook Time: 50 Minutes

Servings: 4

Ingredients

- 2 mild dried chili peppers or 1 to 1 ½ teaspoons chili powder, to taste
- 1 can (15 ounces) diced or crushed tomatoes, fire-roasted if possible
- 2 tablespoons plus 2 teaspoons extra-virgin olive oil
- 1 large yellow or red onion, chopped
- 1 medium red bell pepper, chopped
- ¼ teaspoon fine salt, more to taste
- 4 cloves garlic, pressed or minced
- 2 teaspoons ground cumin
- 2 cans (15 ounces each) black beans, rinsed and drained, or 3 cups cooked black beans
- 4 cups (32 ounces) vegetable broth
- 4 corn tortillas, cut into 2-inch long, ¼-inch-wide strips
- ¼ cup chopped fresh cilantro, divided

- 1 to 2 tablespoons lime juice, to taste

- Freshly ground black pepper, to taste

- Garnish options: Thinly sliced and roughly chopped radish, diced ripe avocado, crumbled feta cheese or drizzle of sour cream

Instructions

1. If using dried chili peppers, toast them in a dry skillet over medium heat or directly over a gas flame with tongs, turning as needed. Toast until fragrant and turning darker all over—this can happen quickly, in just a minute or two. Set aside until the peppers are cool enough to handle, then roughly chop them, discarding the seeds and stem. Combine the canned tomatoes (along with their juices) and chopped peppers in the blender, and blend until smooth. Set aside.

2. In a medium Dutch oven or soup pot, warm 2 tablespoons olive oil over medium heat. Add the onion, bell pepper, and salt. Cook, stirring occasionally, until the onion is tender and turning translucent, about 5 to 7 minutes.

3. Add the garlic and cumin (and chili powder, if using) and cook until fragrant, about 30 seconds to 1 minute. Add the tomato-chili pepper blend (or just plain tomatoes, if going the chili powder route) and cook for a minute, while stirring, to bring out its best flavor.

4. Add the beans and broth, and stir to combine. Raise the mixture to medium-high and bring the mixture to a simmer, then reduce the heat as necessary to maintain a gentle simmer. Simmer for 30 minutes.

5. In the meantime, preheat the oven to 400 degrees Fahrenheit to make the crispy tortilla strips. Line a large, rimmed baking sheet with parchment paper for easy cleanup. On the baking sheet, toss the tortilla strips with the remaining 2 teaspoons olive oil and a sprinkle of salt until lightly and evenly coated. Bake until the strips are crisp and starting to turn golden, about 8 to 12 minutes, tossing halfway. Set aside.

6. Stir most of the cilantro into the soup, reserving a bit for garnish. Stir in 1 tablespoon lime juice. Carefully taste the soup, and add more salt if the flavors don't quite sing (I often add up to ¼ teaspoon salt). Add more lime juice if you'd like a little more zing.

7. Divide the soup into bowls. Top with crispy tortilla strips, the reserved cilantro and any additional

garnishes of your choice. Leftovers will keep well for up to 5 days; rewarm individual servings and top with garnishes when serving. Or freeze individual portions for several months and add toppings after reheating.

Prep Time: 20 Minutes

Cook Time: 15 Minutes

Servings: 2

Ingredients

- 2 tablespoons coconut oil or quality high-heat oil such as avocado oil, divided
- 2 eggs, whisked together with a dash of salt
- 2 big cloves garlic, pressed or minced
- ¾ cup chopped green onions (about 1 bunch)
- Optional: 1 cup chopped vegetables, like bell pepper, carrot or Brussels sprouts
- 1 medium bunch kale (preferably Lacinato but curly green is good, too), ribs removed and leaves chopped
- ¼ teaspoon fine sea salt
- ¾ cup large, unsweetened coconut flakes (not shredded coconut)
- 2 cups cooked and chilled brown rice
- 2 teaspoons reduced-sodium tamari or soy sauce
- 2 teaspoons chili garlic sauce or sriracha
- 1 lime, halved

- Handful fresh cilantro, for garnish

Instructions

1. Heat a large (12-inch or wider) wok, cast iron skillet or non-stick frying pan over medium-high heat. Once the pan is hot enough that a drop of water sizzles on contact, add 1 teaspoon oil and swirl the pan to coat the bottom. Pour in the eggs and cook, stirring frequently, until the eggs are scrambled and lightly set. Transfer the eggs to your empty bowl. Wipe out the pan if necessary with a paper towel (be careful, it's hot!).

2. Add 1 tablespoon oil to the pan and add the garlic, green onions and optional additional vegetables. Cook until fragrant or until the vegetables are tender, stirring frequently, for 30 seconds or longer. Add the kale and salt. Continue to cook until the kale is wilted and tender, stirring frequently, about 1 to 2 minutes. Transfer the contents of the pan to your bowl of eggs.

3. Add the remaining 2 teaspoons oil to the pan. Pour in the coconut flakes and cook, stirring frequently, until the flakes are lightly golden, about 30 seconds. Add the rice to the pan and cook, stirring occasionally,

until the rice is hot, about 3 minutes.

4. Pour the contents of the bowl back into the pan, breaking up the scrambled egg with your spatula or spoon. Once warmed, remove the pan from the heat.

5. Add the tamari, chili garlic sauce and juice of ½ lime. Stir to combine. Taste, and if it's not fantastic yet, add another teaspoon of tamari or a pinch of salt, as needed.

6. Slice the remaining ½ lime into wedges, then divide the fried rice into individual bowls. Garnish with wedges of lime and a sprinkling of torn cilantro leaves, with jars of tamari, chili garlic sauce and/or red pepper flakes on the side, for those who might want more.

Prep Time: 20 Minutes

Cook Time: 45 Minutes

Servings: 6

Ingredients

- 4 tablespoons extra-virgin olive oil, divided
- 1 medium yellow onion, chopped
- 2 medium carrots, peeled and chopped
- 2 medium ribs celery, chopped
- ¼ cup tomato paste
- 2 cups chopped seasonal vegetables (potatoes, yellow squash, zucchini, butternut squash, green beans or peas all work)
- 4 cloves garlic, pressed or minced
- ½ teaspoon dried oregano
- ½ teaspoon dried thyme
- 1 large can (28 ounces) diced tomatoes, with their liquid (or 2 small 15-ounce cans)
- 4 cups (32 ounces) vegetable broth
- 2 cups water
- 1 teaspoon fine sea salt

- 2 bay leaves

- Pinch of red pepper flakes

- Freshly ground black pepper

- 1 cup whole grain orecchiette, elbow or small shell pasta

- 1 can (15 ounces) Great Northern beans or cannellini beans, rinsed and drained, or 1 ½ cups cooked beans

- 2 cups baby spinach, chopped kale or chopped collard greens

- 2 teaspoons lemon juice

- Freshly grated Parmesan cheese, for garnishing (optional)

Instructions

1. Warm 3 tablespoons of the olive oil in a large Dutch oven or stockpot over medium heat. Once the oil is shimmering, add the chopped onion, carrot, celery, tomato paste and a pinch of salt. Cook, stirring often, until the vegetables have softened and the onions are turning translucent, about 7 to 10 minutes.

2. Add the seasonal vegetables, garlic, oregano and thyme. Cook until fragrant while stirring frequently, about 2 minutes.

3. Pour in the diced tomatoes and their juices, broth and water. Add the salt, bay leaves and red pepper flakes. Season generously with freshly ground black pepper.

4. Raise heat to medium-high and bring the mixture to a boil, then partially cover the pot with the lid, leaving about a 1" gap for steam to escape. Reduce heat as necessary to maintain a gentle simmer.

5. Cook for 15 minutes, then remove the lid and add the pasta, beans and greens. Continue simmering, uncovered, for 20 minutes or until the the pasta is cooked al dente and the greens are tender.

6. Remove the pot from the heat, then remove the bay leaves. Stir in the lemon juice and remaining tablespoon of olive oil. Taste and season with more salt (I usually add about ¼ teaspoon more) and pepper until the flavors really sing. Garnish bowls of soup with grated Parmesan, if you'd like.

26. Better Broccoli Casserole

Prep Time: 15 Minutes

Cook Time: 45 Minutes

Servings: 6-8

Ingredients

- 2 cups vegetable broth or water
- 1 cup quinoa (any color), rinsed under running water in a mesh sieve for a minute and drained
- 16 ounces broccoli florets, either pre-packaged or sliced from 2 large bunches of broccoli
- 2 tablespoons olive oil
- ¾ teaspoon salt
- 10 twists of freshly ground black pepper
- ¼ teaspoon red pepper flakes, omit if sensitive to spice
- 8 ounces (about 2 ½ cups) freshly grated cheddar cheese, divided
- 1 cup low-fat milk (cow's milk tastes best but unsweetened plain almond milk works, too)
- ½ tablespoon butter or 1 ½ teaspoons olive oil
- 1 clove garlic, pressed or minced

- 1 slice whole wheat bread (substitute gluten-free bread for a gluten-free casserole)

Instructions

1. Preheat oven to 400 degrees Fahrenheit. Line a large, rimmed baking sheet with parchment paper for easy cleanup.
2. To cook the quinoa: Bring the vegetable broth or water to boil in a heavy-bottomed, medium-sized pot. Add the quinoa, reduce heat to low and simmer, uncovered, for 17 to 20 minutes, or until all of the liquid is absorbed. Cover and set aside to steam for 10 minutes.
3. To roast the broccoli: Slice any large broccoli florets in half to make bite-sized pieces. Transfer the broccoli to your prepared baking sheet and toss with 2 tablespoons olive oil, until lightly coated on all sides. Sprinkle with salt and arrange in a single layer. Bake for about 20 minutes, until the broccoli is tender and starting to caramelize on the edges.
4. To make the breadcrumbs: Tear your piece of bread into bite-sized pieces and toss them into a food processor or blender. Process until the bread has

broken into small crumbs. In a small pan over medium heat, melt the butter. Add the garlic and cook just until fragrant, stirring often. Add the bread crumbs and cook for 2 to 3 minutes, until slightly browned and crisp. Set aside to cool. (If you cooked your bread crumbs in a cast iron skillet, transfer them to a bowl to prevent them from burning.)

5. Reduce the oven heat to 350 degrees. Add the salt, pepper and red pepper flakes to the pot of quinoa, and stir to combine. Set aside ¾ cup of the cheese for later, then add the rest of the cheese to the pot. Pour in the milk and stir until the cheese and milk are evenly incorporated in the quinoa.

6. Pour the cheesy quinoa into a 9-inch square baking dish and top with the roasted broccoli. Stir until the broccoli is evenly mixed in with the quinoa. Sprinkle the surface of the casserole with the reserved ¾ cup cheese, then sprinkle the breadcrumbs on top.

7. Bake, uncovered, for 25 minutes, until the top is golden. Allow to cool for 10 minutes before serving.

Prep Time: 20 Minutes

Cook Time: 15 Minutes

Servings: 2-3

Ingredients

- 1 ½ teaspoons + 2 tablespoons avocado oil or safflower oil, divided
- 2 eggs, whisked together
- 1 small white onion, finely chopped (about 1 cup)
- 2 medium carrots, finely chopped (about ½ cup)
- 2 cups additional veggies, cut into very small pieces for quick cooking (options include snow peas, asparagus, broccoli, cabbage, bell pepper, and/or fresh or frozen peas—no need to thaw first)
- ¼ teaspoon salt, more to taste
- 1 tablespoon grated or finely minced fresh ginger
- 2 large cloves garlic, pressed or minced
- Pinch of red pepper flakes
- 2 cups cooked brown rice
- 1 cup greens (optional), such as spinach, baby kale or tatsoi

- 3 green onions, chopped

- 1 tablespoon reduced-sodium tamari or soy sauce

- 1 teaspoon toasted sesame oil

- Chili-garlic sauce or sriracha, for serving (optional)

Instructions

1. This recipe comes together quickly. Before you get started, make sure that all of your ingredients are prepped and within an arm's reach from the stove. Also have an empty bowl nearby for holding the cooked eggs and veggies. I'm suggesting that you start over medium-high heat, but if at any point you catch a whiff of oil or food burning, reduce the heat to medium.

2. Warm a large cast iron or stainless steel skillet over medium-high heat until a few drops of water evaporate within a couple of seconds. Immediately add 1 ½ teaspoons of oil and swirl the pan to coat the bottom. Add the scrambled eggs and swirl the pan so they cover the bottom. Cook until they are just lightly set, flipping or stirring along the way. Transfer the eggs to a bowl and wipe out the pan with a heat-proof spatula.

3. Return the pan to heat and add 1 tablespoon of oil. Add the onion and carrots and cook, stirring often, until the onions are translucent and the carrots are tender, about 3 to 5 minutes.

4. Add the remaining veggies and salt. Continue cooking, stirring occasionally (don't stir too often, or the veggies won't have a chance to turn golden on the edges), until the veggies are cooked through and turning golden, about 3 to 5 more minutes. In the meantime, use the edge of your spatula or a spoon to break up the scrambled eggs into smaller pieces.

5. Use a big spatula or spoon to transfer the contents of the pan to the bowl with the cooked eggs. Return the pan to heat and the remaining 1 tablespoon oil. Add the ginger, garlic and red pepper flakes, and cook until fragrant while stirring constantly, about 30 seconds. Add the rice and mix it all together. Cook, stirring occasionally, until the rice is hot and starting to turn golden on the edges, about 3 to 5 minutes.

6. Add the greens (if using) and green onions, and stir to combine. Add the cooked veggies and eggs and stir to combine. Remove the pan from the heat and stir in the tamari and sesame oil. Taste, and add a little more tamari if you'd like more soy flavor (don't overdo it or

it will drown out the other flavors) or salt, if the dish needs an extra boost of overall flavor.

7. Divide into bowls and serve immediately. I usually serve mine with chili-garlic sauce or sriracha on the side. Leftovers store well in the refrigerator, covered, for 3 to 4 days (if you used purple cabbage, it might stain your scrambled eggs a funny blue color, but it's fine to eat).

Prep Time: 10 Minutes

Cook Time: 45 Minutes

Servings: 6

Ingredients

- 2 tablespoons extra-virgin olive oil
- 2 medium yellow onions, chopped
- 3 celery ribs, finely chopped
- 1 large carrot, peeled and sliced into thin rounds
- 6 garlic cloves, pressed or minced
- 4 ½ teaspoons ground cumin
- ½ teaspoon red pepper flakes (use ¼ teaspoon if you're sensitive to spice)
- 4 cans (15 ounces each) black beans, rinsed and drained
- 4 cups (32 ounces) low-sodium vegetable broth
- ¼ cup chopped fresh cilantro (optional)
- 1 to 2 teaspoons sherry vinegar, to taste, or 2 tablespoons fresh lime juice
- Sea salt and freshly ground black pepper, to taste

- Optional garnishes: diced avocado, extra cilantro, thinly sliced radishes, tortilla chips...

Instructions

1. Heat the olive oil in a large Dutch oven or soup pot over medium heat until shimmering. Add the onions, celery and carrot and a light sprinkle of salt. Cook, stirring occasionally, until the vegetable are soft, about 10 to 15 minutes.

2. Stir in the garlic, cumin and red pepper flakes and cook until fragrant, about 30 seconds. Pour in the beans and broth and bring to a simmer over medium-high heat. Cook, reducing heat as necessary to maintain a gentle simmer, until the broth is flavorful and the beans are very tender, about 30 minutes.

3. Transfer about 4 cups of the soup to a stand blender, securely fasten the lid, and blend until smooth (never fill your blender past the maximum fill line, and beware the steam that escapes from the top of the blender, it's very hot). Or, use an immersion blender to blend a portion of the soup.

4. Return the pureed soup to the pot, stir in the cilantro, vinegar/lime juice and salt and pepper, to taste. Serve.

Prep Time: 10 Minutes

Cook Time: 10 Minutes

Servings: 2

Ingredients

- 8 ounces fresh collard greens (about 10 big leaves)
- ⅓ or more of a package of whole wheat thin spaghetti or "spaghettini"
- 3 tablespoons pine nuts
- olive oil (the good stuff)
- 2 small cloves garlic, pressed
- big pinch red pepper flakes
- sea salt and black pepper
- 1 ounce Parmesan cheese
- ½ or more of a lemon, cut into wedges

Instructions

1. Bring a big pot of salted water to a boil and cook the pasta according to directions. Drain quickly, reserving a bit of cooking water, and set aside.

2. Cut out the center rib of each collard green. Stack a few greens at a time and roll them up into a cigar-like shape. Slice across the roll as thinly as possible (⅛″ to ¼″). Shake up the greens and give them a few chops so the strands aren't so long.

3. Heat a heavy-bottomed 12″ skillet over medium heat and toast the pine nuts until they start to turn golden and fragrant. Pour them out of the skillet and save for later.

4. Return the skillet to medium heat and pour in a tablespoon of olive oil. Sprinkle in a big pinch of red pepper flakes and the garlic and stir. Once the oil is hot enough to shimmer, toss in all of your collard greens. Sprinkle the greens with salt. Stirring often (try not to let them clump), sauté the greens for about three minutes.

5. Remove the pan from heat. Scoop the greens into the pasta pot and toss with another drizzle of olive oil, adding pasta water if necessary. Divide onto plates, top with pine nuts and Parmesan shavings and serve with two big lemon wedges per person.

Prep Time: 10 Minutes

Cook Time: 30 Minutes

Servings: 4

Ingredients

- 1 ¼ cups brown jasmine rice or long-grain brown rice, rinsed
- 1 tablespoon coconut oil or olive oil
- 1 small white onion, chopped (about 1 cup)
- Pinch of salt, more to taste
- 1 tablespoon finely grated fresh ginger (about a 1-inch nub of ginger)
- 2 cloves garlic, pressed or minced
- 1 red bell pepper, sliced into thin 2-inch long strips
- 1 yellow, orange or green bell pepper, sliced into thin 2-inch long strips
- 3 carrots, peeled and sliced on the diagonal into ¼-inch thick rounds (about 1 cup)
- 2 tablespoons Thai red curry paste
- 1 can (14 ounces) regular coconut milk
- ½ cup water

- 1 ½ cups packed thinly sliced kale (tough ribs removed first), preferably the Tuscan/lacinato/dinosaur variety
- 1 ½ teaspoons coconut sugar or turbinado (raw) sugar or brown sugar
- 1 tablespoon tamari or soy sauce
- 2 teaspoons rice vinegar or fresh lime juice
- Garnishes/sides: handful of chopped fresh basil or cilantro, optional red pepper flakes, optional sriracha or chili garlic sauce

Instructions

1. To cook the rice, bring a large pot of water to boil. Add the rinsed rice and continue boiling for 30 minutes, reducing heat as necessary to prevent overflow. Remove from heat, drain the rice and return the rice to pot. Cover and let the rice rest for 10 minutes or longer, until you're ready to serve. Just before serving, season the rice to taste with salt and fluff it with a fork.

2. To make the curry, warm a large skillet with deep sides over medium heat. Once it's hot, add the oil. Add the onion and a sprinkle of salt and cook, stirring

often, until the onion has softened and is turning translucent, about 5 minutes. Add the ginger and garlic and cook until fragrant, about 30 seconds, while stirring continuously.

3. Add the bell peppers and carrots. Cook until the bell peppers are fork-tender, 3 to 5 more minutes, stirring occasionally. Then add the curry paste and cook, stirring often, for 2 minutes.

4. Add the coconut milk, water, kale and sugar, and stir to combine. Bring the mixture to a simmer over medium heat. Reduce heat as necessary to maintain a gentle simmer and cook until the peppers, carrots and kale have softened to your liking, about 5 to 10 minutes, stirring occasionally.

5. Remove the pot from the heat and season with tamari and rice vinegar. Add salt (I added ¼ teaspoon for optimal flavor), to taste. If the curry needs a little more punch, add ½ teaspoon more tamari, or for more acidity, add ½ teaspoon more rice vinegar. Divide rice and curry into bowls and garnish with chopped cilantro and a sprinkle of red pepper flakes, if you'd like. If you love spicy curries, serve with sriracha or chili garlic sauce on the side.

www.ingramcontent.com/pod-product-compliance
Lightning Source LLC
Chambersburg PA
CBHW061920270726
48658CB00005BB/1715